# UNDERSTANDING

# HERBAL

# MEDICINE

## Unlocking The Power Of Nature For Key Principles For Holistic Healing, Focus Strategies, Achieving Optimal Health, Natural Healing And More

## DR. KARSON BRYAN

# DISCLAIMER

This book's content is meant to be used solely for general informative purposes. Despite having taken every precaution to guarantee the content's accuracy, the author disclaims all duty and responsibility for any errors or omissions. It is recommended that readers exercise caution and, if needed, seek expert guidance. Any and all liability for losses, damages, or other outcomes arising from the use of the material included in this book is disclaimed by the author and publisher. All referenced product names and trademarks are the property of their respective owners and are merely cited for identification. Any likeness to real people or things is entirely accidental. Since it is a work of fiction, this book should not be used as a substitute for professional, legal, or medical advice. It is advised that readers seek advice on particular issues from qualified experts."

Please make sure that this disclaimer is modified to fit the particular requirements and subject matter of your book. Seeking advice from a legal expert is also a smart option if you have any questions or require a more thorough disclaimer for your specific book.

# TABLE OF CONTENTS

# CHAPTER ONE

# HERBAL MEDICINE

## INTRODUCTION

### HERBAL MEDICINE: AN ART AND SCIENCE

Herbal medicine combines factual knowledge, traditional wisdom, and contemporary scientific understanding to create a blend of art and science. The traditional knowledge and age-old methods that have been handed down through the generations are all included in the art of herbal medicine. It entails the deft selection and processing of herbs, the creation of cures, and the intuitive knowledge of the physiological effects of herbs. This art frequently conveys a rich tapestry of rituals and symbols and is firmly anchored in cultural traditions. Conversely, the study of herbal medicine explores the molecular makeup of plants, their pharmacological characteristics, and how they affect human physiology. It calls for an in-depth knowledge of photochemistry, botany, and the scientific techniques utilized in the study of medicinal plants. Herbal medicine is built on the synergy between art and science, which enables the creation of evidence-based practices as well as the preservation of traditional remedies.

## THE ORIGINS OF HERBAL MEDICINE IN HISTORY

Herbal medicine has a long history that is intricately linked to the advancement of human civilization. Throughout human history, humans have looked to plants for both healing and nutrition. Herbal knowledge was transmitted orally and documented in ancient writings. Many of the herbal medicines used by ancient civilizations including the Sumerians, Egyptians, Greeks, and Chinese are still in use today. The history of herbal medicine has been profoundly impacted by the writings of individuals such as Dioscorides, Hippocrates, and Shen Nong. These historical foundations still have an impact on contemporary herbalism, offering a wealth of customs, expertise, and insight to draw from.

## MODERN RESURRECTION OF HERBAL MEDICINE

Herbal medicine has experienced a notable resurgence in acceptance and appeal in the last few decades. The efficacy of many herbal medicines has been validated by scientific research, and developments in science have also contributed to this renaissance. Other factors include a renewed appreciation for traditional wisdom and a growing interest in natural and holistic approaches to health. Herbal treatment is experiencing a modern renaissance that goes beyond a throwback to include the incorporation of herbal medicine into conventional medical practices. To offer patients with complete care, herbalists collaborate with medical specialists and utilize herbal therapies in addition to conventional therapy. Herbal therapy has become more popular as a result of the trend towards sustainability and environmental consciousness, which has driven people to look for all-natural remedies that are not harmful to the environment.

The goal of this book is to provide a thorough examination of the field of herbal medicine, covering both its art and science. With its examination of the historical foundations of herbal medicine and its contemporary resurgence, it offers readers a comprehensive grasp of this age-old and developing discipline. We will explore the cutting-edge advancements in modern herbal medicine as well as the ageless wisdom of herbal traditions across the book's pages, giving readers the knowledge and skills they need to take advantage of plants' healing powers in their own lives.

# CHAPTER TWO

# KNOWLEDGE OF HERBAL MEDICINE

## WHAT ARE HERBS AND HERBAL MEDICINE?

Herbs are plants or plant parts leaves, roots, flowers, and seeds, for example that have been used for their fragrant, culinary, and medicinal uses for ages. The use of these plants and their extracts to prevent, treat, or mitigate certain health disorders is known as herbal medicine, phototherapy, or botanical medicine. It is a natural and holistic approach to healthcare that makes use of nature's healing powers. Herbs have been used for medical purposes since the dawn of civilization, and they are still an essential component of both conventional medical practices and contemporary complementary and alternative therapies.

# THE FUNDAMENTALS OF HERBAL MEDICINE

Numerous basic concepts guide herbal healing. Herbs are utilized to promote and encourage the body's natural healing process since it first and foremost acknowledges the body's fundamental ability to heal itself. The idea of vitalism, which emphasizes the importance of vital life energies in preserving health, is one that herbalists frequently consider. They think that by nourishing and balancing these essential factors, herbs might enhance general well-being. Herbal medicine also follows the tenet of customized care, in which an herbalist creates a remedy based on the unique needs and constitution of each patient. Effective herbal medicine is not a one-size-fits-all solution, and thorough assessment and diagnosis are essential.

# A HOLISTIC PERSPECTIVE ON HEALTH

Herbal medicine takes a holistic approach to health, acknowledging that a person's physical, emotional, and environmental conditions are just a few of the interrelated components that affect their overall health. Instead of focusing only on treating symptoms, it aims to address the underlying causes of health problems. In addition to herbal medicines, holistic herbalists stress the significance of diet, lifestyle, and emotional well-being. Rather than concentrating only on one symptom or illness, this all-encompassing approach seeks to restore harmony and balance to the whole person. Herbalists strive to support not just physical healing but also emotional and mental well-being, taking into account the mind-body link and the negative effects of stress on health.

# CONVENTIONAL HERBAL MEDICINE SYSTEMS

With a long history, herbal medicine is ingrained in many traditional healing practices all around the world. These systems include Indigenous medical practices, Indian Ayurveda, Traditional Chinese Medicine (TCM), and many more. Every tradition has its own set of tenets, herbal medicines, and diagnostic techniques that have been passed down through the decades. For example, Ayurveda divides people into several doshas according to their constitution and utilizes herbs to balance these energies, whereas TCM emphasizes the idea of yin and yang and the flow of qi (energy). Herbal medicine systems with a long history provide a lot of information and expertise about the use of plants in treatment.

# COMBINING TRADITIONAL MEDICAL PRACTICES WITH HERBAL MEDICINE

These days, there's a rising interest in combining traditional therapy with herbal medicine. This integrative method acknowledges that each system has advantages and disadvantages and that they might work in concert to deliver more thorough patient care. A lot of medical professionals are willing to talk to their patients about herbal medicines, and studies are being done to find out how safe and effective different plants are. To prevent any interactions or negative consequences, it is crucial to make sure that any integration is carried out under competent supervision and knowledge. It is advised that patients disclose to their healthcare practitioners any use of herbal remedies.

Using plants and their extracts to promote health and treat a variety of ailments is a time-honored technique known as herbal medicine. It is based on the ideas of personalized care, natural healing, and a holistic approach to wellness. Herbal medicine's traditional systems provide insightful information, and as the potential advantages of this method become apparent, the integration of herbal therapy with traditional healthcare is growing in popularity. For individuals looking for complementary and alternative therapies, herbal medicine continues to play a vital part in the diversified landscape of healthcare by providing a natural and all-encompassing alternative.

# CHAPTER THREE

## THE DOMAIN OF REMEDY PLANTS

### RECOGNIZING AND OBTAINING THERAPEUTIC PLANTS

Herbalism and traditional medicine rely heavily on the identification and procurement of therapeutic plants. Due to their healing qualities, medicinal plants have been utilized for ages in many different cultures throughout the world. To guarantee the safety and effectiveness of these plants in herbal treatments, proper identification is essential. It combines an understanding of plants, close observation, and occasionally even chemical analysis. Experts, herbalists, and botanical guides are essential in helping people discover and get therapeutic plants. This information is frequently passed down through the generations, maintaining the conventional wisdom surrounding plant identification.

# GROWING AND TAKING CARE OF MEDICINAL HERBS

Growing and cultivating medicinal herbs is a sustainable way to guarantee a steady supply of these priceless plants. Greater control over the type, amount, and sustainability of sources of therapeutic plants is made possible by cultivation. Additionally, it lessens the strain on untamed populations, which may be susceptible to overharvesting. Depending on the particular needs of each plant, gardens, fields, or greenhouses can be used for the growth of medicinal herbs. To provide these herbs with the best growing conditions possible, factors including soil quality, climate, and water availability must be carefully taken into account.

## ETHICAL HARVESTING AND WILDCRAFTING

Another way to obtain these priceless botanicals is through the practice of "wild crafting," which is the process of gathering therapeutic plants from their native environments. Wild crafting, however, needs to be done extremely carefully and environmentally conscious. For wild plant populations to remain healthy and abundant, ethical gathering techniques are crucial. The fundamentals of sustainable foraging, such as avoiding overharvesting, honoring the seasonal and reproductive cycles of plants, and reducing ecological effects, should be thoroughly understood by harvesters. A thorough awareness of ecosystems and the delicate balance of nature is necessary for proper wild crafting.

## ECO-FRIENDLY METHODS FOR HERBAL AGRICULTURE

To protect the integrity of sources of medicinal plants for future generations, sustainable agricultural practices are essential in the herbal industry. These methods seek to increase biodiversity, lessen the negative effects of farming on the environment, and utilize less toxic chemicals. To establish sustainable herbal farms, methods such as organic farming, permaculture, and agroforestry can be utilized. Moreover, natural pest management techniques, companion planting, and crop rotation support the upkeep of robust and healthy ecosystems on these farms.

Herbal gardening that uses sustainable methods benefits not just the surrounding ecosystems but also the medicinal plants themselves. These methods save water supplies, promote pollinators and other beneficial species, and improve the quality of the land. The larger objectives of environmental preservation and a holistic approach to health and wellness are compatible with sustainable herbal growing.

A crucial first step in the field of herbalism and traditional medicine is recognizing and obtaining therapeutic plants. Ensuring a sustained supply of these precious plants requires both ethical wild crafting and the cultivation of medical herbs.

# CHAPTER FOUR

# MAKING HERBAL MEDICINES

## GATHERING AND DESICCATING HERBS

These are essential processes in the making of herbal medicines. The quality and potency of the plants used in herbal remedies are guaranteed by using proper harvesting techniques. Typically, herbs are gathered at the height of their growth season, when the majority of their therapeutic qualities are present. Selecting the ideal time of day is crucial; this is typically in the morning when the plants are clear of dew and before the heat of the sun evaporates volatile oils. For optimal efficacy, herbs are best gathered before they blossom.

Drying the herbs comes next after harvesting. By preserving the herbs through drying, mold, and deterioration are avoided while the medicinal qualities are retained. Herbs can be dried by hanging them in bunches in a well-ventilated place, letting them air dry, or using a low-temperature dehydrator. To preserve their effectiveness, the dried herbs should be kept out of direct sunlight and dampened in sealed containers.

## METHODS FOR HERBAL EXTRACTION

Extracting the active ingredients from herbs to make herbal medicines is known as herbal extraction. Different types of herbs and applications can benefit from different extraction techniques. Cold pressing, percolation, and maceration are a few popular extraction techniques. Herbs are macerated—that is, they are soaked in a liquid, usually oil or alcohol—to gradually extract their medicinal ingredients. The more involved process of percolation, which is frequently used to make tinctures, extracts ingredients by pressure or gravity. Aromatic herbs are cold-pressed to extract essential oils.

# DECOCTIONS & INFUSIONS

These age-old, straightforward techniques are used to draw therapeutic qualities from herbs. Similar to brewing tea, infusions are created by covering fresh or dried herbs with boiling water and letting them simmer. Conversely, harder plant parts like bark or roots are boiled to extract their therapeutic chemicals to make decoctions. Herbal teas prepared using these techniques can be drank for several health advantages, such as easing digestion and encouraging relaxation.

## TINCTURES

Typically produced with glycerin or alcohol as the solvent, tinctures are concentrated liquid extracts of herbs. Tinctures' lengthy shelf life and simplicity of usage make them highly valued. Certain tinctures have a high alcohol level that facilitates convenient administration while preserving the botanical characteristics. Herbs can be macerated in a selected solvent for a long time to create tinctures, which have a variety of uses, including topical and oral use.

## HERBAL OILS AND SALVES

The process of creating herbal oils and salves involves infusing herbs into waxes or carrier oils, respectively. To extract the therapeutic properties of fresh or dried herbs, the oil or wax is heated. These formulations can be used topically on the skin to nourish it, heal wounds, and ease aching muscles, among other things. Almond oil, coconut oil, and olive oil are common carrier oils for herbal infusions.

## HERBAL TEAS AND BREWS

Among the most widely used and recognizable types of herbal treatments are herbal teas and brews. They are created by steeping herbs in hot water, and people drink them for their tasty and therapeutic properties. Herbal teas can be made with specific health objectives in mind, such as enhancing immunity or relieving anxiety. Ginger, peppermint, and chamomile are popular plants for teas. Similar to teas, brews are made using a mixture of herbs and additional components, such as spices or honey, providing a more personalized method of using herbal medicines.

Creating herbal treatments requires a thorough understanding of harvesting, drying, and several extraction techniques. These essential stages determine the potency and quality of your herbal remedies, whether you're creating tinctures, oils, salves, or teas. Making herbal remedies with the right method and care guarantees that you'll be able to fully utilize nature's therapeutic power.

# CHAPTER FIVE

# PUTTING TOGETHER YOUR HERBAL MEDICINE SUPPLY

## ESSENTIAL TOOLS AND EQUIPMENT

Having the appropriate tools and equipment at the outset is crucial to creating an herbal medicine toolkit that works. The main things you'll require are:

1. A mortar and pestle is a necessary tool for the efficient grinding and mixing of herbs, which enables you to make tinctures, salves, and herbal treatments. Opting for a material that aligns with your tastes is crucial, as they are available in wood, ceramic, or stone varieties.

2. Herb Scissors or Shears: These specialized tools are made to cut herbs accurately, which simplifies the process of preparing herbs for infusions, decoctions, and teas.

3. Glass Jars & Bottles: Since glass doesn't react with herbs and preserves the integrity of your concoctions, it's the recommended material for storing herbal remedies. For tinctures, oils, and salves, different sizes come in helpful.

4. Cheesecloths and strainers are necessary to ensure that your preparations are free of plant debris when filtering herbal infusions. Using cheesecloth and a fine-mesh strainer will assist you in getting the right level of clarity from your herbal drinks.

5. Digital Scale: A digital scale is very helpful for precisely measuring herbal components, particularly for creating tinctures or salves. This guarantees your herbal preparations are consistent.

6. Labels and Markers: For organization and safety, make sure your herbal remedies are properly labeled. Add the name of the plant, the

date of preparation, and any special directions for using it.

7. Use herb identification books or apps to make sure you choose the right herbs for your cures by accurately identifying herbs and their qualities.

## PUTTING TOGETHER YOUR HERBAL FIRST AID KIT

Having medicines for common illnesses close at hand is a practical method to create a herbal first aid kit. Add the following things:

• Sterile dressings and bandages: these are necessary for the treatment of wounds.

• Antiseptic Herbs: Wounds can be cleaned and disinfected using calendula, plantain, and yarrow.

• Aloe Vera Gel: A calming treatment for skin irritations and burns.

• Herbal Tinctures: Include tinctures such as arnica for pain treatment and Echinacea for immune system support in your bag.

• Herbal Salves: Cuts, bruises, and small burns can be treated with calendula or comfrey salves.

• Herbal Teas: Teas with chamomile and peppermint are great for soothing stomach problems and promoting relaxation.

• Essential Oils: Tea tree and lavender oils are useful for skin care and aromatherapy.

• Insect Repellent: To ward off insects, make your own or buy a herbal repellent.

## HERBAL TREATMENTS FOR TYPICAL ILLNESSES

1. Cold and Flu: Herbs such as elderberry, Echinacea, and ginger can help you combat colds and flu. Echinacea has anti-inflammatory and anti-illness effects, while elderberry syrup is well known for strengthening the immune system. Nausea and congestion can be relieved with ginger tea or pills.

2. Digestive Problems: Fennel, ginger, and peppermint are popular herbs for digestive issues. Ginger helps calm troubled tummies, and peppermint tea relieves indigestion and bloating. Both adults and children with colic and gas can benefit from fennel tea.

3. Skin Conditions: Lavender, calendula, and aloe vera are great herbs for a variety of skin issues. Aloe vera is a home cure for sunburn and skin irritations, and calendula salve or cream helps relieve dry, itchy skin and small wounds. Because of its calming and antibacterial qualities, lavender essential oil can be diluted and applied topically.

4. Herbs that are recognized to be calming, such as lavender, chamomile, and valerian, are effective in reducing stress and anxiety. Valerian tea is beneficial for anxiety and sleep issues, while chamomile tea is a popular choice for relaxation. Aromatherapy can employ lavender essential oil to promote calmness and lessen stress.

5. Pain and Inflammation: Herbs like arnica, turmeric, and willow bark may be used to treat pain and inflammation. An all-natural treatment for bruises and sore muscles is arnica oil or salve. Turmeric can be used in cooking or as a supplement because of its anti-inflammatory qualities. Willow bark has a natural aspirin precursor called salicin, which is useful for treating minor discomfort.

By incorporating these ideas into your herbal medicine toolkit, you may treat a variety of common illnesses and promote well-being and health naturally. When taking herbal medicines, especially for more serious health conditions, never forget to get advice and customized suggestions from a healthcare practitioner or herbalist.

# CHAPTER SIX

# HERBAL TREATMENT AND WELL-BEING

## ENCOURAGING OPTIMAL HEALTH WITH HERBS

With a millennium of history, herbal medicine is a well-liked and successful method of encouraging overall health and well-being. Because of their therapeutic qualities, herbs have been used by many civilizations all over the world. They are essential to the body's ability to remain balanced and vibrant. You can address a variety of health issues and promote your general well-being by including herbs in your daily routine. The natural, all-encompassing approach to health that herbs offer emphasizes the body's capacity to cure itself with the correct resources and assistance.

# HERBAL ADAPTOGENS AND TONICS

For preserving and regaining vitality, herbal medicine must include both types of herbs. Herbal tonics are concoctions made from plants that are intended to energize and fortify the body. They are frequently used regularly to support overall wellness and fend off sickness. Conversely, a certain class of herbs known as adaptogens aids in the body's ability to adjust to stress and preserve equilibrium. They are highly valued because they can strengthen the body's defenses against mental and physical pressures. Adaptogens, such as ginseng, Rhodiola, and ashwagandha, can be very useful in assisting the body in meeting the demands of contemporary living.

## DETOXIFICATION AND CLEANING

For the body to eliminate accumulated toxins and preserve maximum health, detoxification, and cleansing are necessary procedures. Herbs are quite important in helping these processes. Herbs that help the liver detoxify the body include burdock root, milk thistle, and dandelion. Herbs that are used for cleansing, such as aloe vera and psyllium husk, aid in removing waste and toxins from the digestive system. By including these herbs in your diet, you can help your body become purified and feel more balanced.

## IMMUNE SYSTEM SUPPORT WITH HERBS

Using herbs to support the immune system is a healthy and efficient alternative. Herbs that support the immune system, such as Echinacea, astragalus, and elderberry, are well known for strengthening the body's defenses against infections. These herbs can be used in times of increased susceptibility to infections or daily to help avoid disease. Herbal assistance can be an invaluable complement to your wellness routine in a world where immunity maintenance is critical.

# IMPROVING MENTAL FOCUS AND CLARITY

Both general well-being and productivity depend on mental focus and clarity. Herbs have the potential to improve focus and cognitive performance. For instance, ginkgo biloba is well known for enhancing memory and cognitive function. Furthermore, herbs with a reputation for promoting mental clarity and lowering stress include gotu kola and bacopa. You can have a clearer, more concentrated mind and enhanced cognitive performance by including these herbs in your everyday regimen.

Herbal medicine is a comprehensive and tried-and-true strategy for fostering the best possible health and well-being. You can use the power of nature to assist your health by including immune system support, detoxification techniques, mental clarity, and focus herbs, adaptogens, and herbal tonics into your lifestyle.

# CHAPTER SEVEN

# HERBAL TREATMENT FOR PARTICULAR ILLNESSES

## RESPIRATORY HEALTH

Respiratory health is an important element of total well-being, and herbal therapy has been applied for millennia to address various respiratory problems. Herbs like Eucalyptus, Thyme, and Licorice have proved their effectiveness in calming coughs and reducing congestion. For example, eucalyptus includes chemicals that can aid in clearing respiratory discomfort and opening airways. Due to its antispasmodic qualities, thyme is frequently utilized in herbal treatments for respiratory conditions including bronchitis.

## CARDIOVASCULAR HEALTH

Living a long and active life requires maintaining a healthy cardiovascular system. One important factor in supporting cardiovascular health is herbal medicine. Hawthorn has been a staple of traditional herbal treatments for ages due to its well-known heart-supporting properties. Another herb with cardiovascular advantages is garlic, which also helps lower cholesterol and high blood pressure. Herbs with anti-inflammatory qualities, such as ginger and turmeric, may also improve general heart health.

## WOMEN'S HEALTH

A plethora of therapies tailored specifically to address women's health issues are available through herbal medicine. Menstrual cycle regulation and menopausal symptoms have been treated with herbs including chaste tree and black cohosh. Rich in phytoestrogens, red clover can aid with hormone regulation. Moreover, raspberry leaf is frequently advised throughout pregnancy to facilitate a more comfortable delivery by strengthening the uterine muscles.

These herbs can be quite helpful in treating women's health problems in a more all-natural way.

## MEN'S HEALTH

Herbal medicines can also be beneficial for men's health issues. For instance, saw palmetto is widely used to promote prostate health and ease the symptoms of benign prostatic hyperplasia (BPH). Ginseng has been shown to give men more energy and general well-being. Another plant that can be used to treat diseases like an enlarged prostate is nettle root. An all-natural method of treating men's health problems is provided by these herbal remedies.

## YOUNGSTERS AND HERBAL REMEDIES

Herbal remedies should be used carefully and cautiously when dealing with youngsters. Some herbs, like chamomile and ginger, are safe for kids and can ease common problems including upset stomachs, colic, and discomfort associated with teething. Nonetheless, it's imperative to speak with a medical expert or herbalist before administering herbal treatments to children. It's important to carefully alter dosages and preparations to protect children's health and safety.

## ELDERLY AND HERBAL CARE

As people age, they may experience a variety of health issues. Herbal medicine can be a helpful tool in managing these issues. Herbs known to be adaptogenic, such as Rhodiola and ashwagandha, can help lower stress and boost energy. Ginkgo biloba is frequently used to help older adults with their memory and cognitive function. Additionally, age-related joint pain and inflammation may be relieved by herbs like boswellia and turmeric. When employing herbal medicines in the older population, it's important to take into account specific medical conditions and possible drug interactions.

Herbal medicine provides a wide range of treatments for certain medical issues, such as cardiovascular, respiratory, women's, men's, children's, and senior care. Herbs can offer safe, all-natural alternatives to conventional medicines, but it's important to speak with medical professionals or herbalists to be sure the right quantities and usage is being followed, particularly for older and fragile populations like children. Including herbal treatments in one's medical regimen can be a beneficial and complementary strategy for reaching and preserving maximum health.

# CHAPTER EIGHT

# HERBAL TREATMENTS AND DIETARY PLANS

## HERBAL SUPPLEMENTS & DIETARY SUPPORT

For ages, herbal supplements have been a vital component of traditional medical systems across the globe. In the field of contemporary healthcare, their acceptance is only growing. These supplements cover a broad spectrum of plant-based goods that are taken to support health and well-being, such as tinctures, powders, and botanical extracts. Supplements containing herbs are frequently used to supplement diets and treat particular medical conditions. They provide a complete, all-natural method for preserving and enhancing general health. The ability of herbal supplements to supply vital nutrients and bioactive substances that may be absent from a person's regular diet is one of their main benefits.

Numerous health advantages, including immunological support, stress reduction, and digestive health, can be obtained from herbal supplements. Well-known examples are ginkgo biloba for cognitive function, turmeric for anti-inflammatory effects, and Echinacea for immunological support. Herbs that help induce calm and reduce anxiety include valerian and chamomile. Herbal supplements can combine with drugs and have specific effects, so it's important to use them carefully and under a doctor's supervision.

## HERBAL COOKING AND CULINARY HERBS

Using herbs in food preparation has a long history in human civilization and has developed into an art form that improves food flavor while also benefiting human health and well-being. Culinary herbs come in a variety of flavors, textures, and scents and are frequently grown in home gardens or kitchens across the globe.

These herbs include mint, oregano, rosemary, basil, thyme, and many more. Culinary herbs enhance our meals with multiple nutritional advantages in addition to their delicious flavors.

Essential vitamins, minerals, and antioxidants found in culinary herbs can help with several health issues. For instance, vitamin K, which is necessary for blood clotting and bone health, is found in basil, while antioxidants found in rosemary help shield cells from harm. A meal's nutritional worth can be increased by adding fresh herbs to it without using a lot of calories or salt. Herbs' vivid hues and fragrant scents can also pique appetites, enhancing the flavor and satisfaction of food.

Cooking with culinary herbs regularly improves the taste of food and encourages a healthier diet. They can be included in a wide range of dishes, including salads, soups, entrées, and desserts. Cooking with herbs creates a world of taste sensations and culinary adventures that make eating healthily pleasurable and long-lasting.

The concept of mixing specific nutrients from herbs and other food sources to generate a harmonious, health-promoting effect on the body is known as "nutritional synergy with herbs." Compared to when these components are ingested separately, this synergy can improve the absorption and utilization of vital nutrients and bioactive substances, leading to greater health benefits.

Iron-rich herbs like parsley and vitamin C-rich fruits like oranges, for instance, can enhance the body's absorption of iron, which makes them a useful combo for preventing iron deficiency anemia. Likewise, combining turmeric, which has curcumin, with black pepper, which has piperine, increases curcumin's bioavailability and optimizes its antioxidant and anti-inflammatory effects.

Herbs' nutritional synergy can also aid in a meal's macronutrient balance. Incorporating herbs like fenugreek or cinnamon into meals high in carbohydrates can help control blood sugar levels. Better glycemic management is encouraged by this combination, which may help those who have diabetes or want to have consistent energy levels all day.

To sum up, nutritional synergy with herbs, culinary herbs, and herbal supplements all play important roles in promoting our health and well-being. Herbs can be incorporated into a well-balanced diet, taken as nutritional supplements, or used as flavor enhancers in cooking to support a holistic approach to maintaining a healthy lifestyle and preventing various health conditions. Investigating these ideas is crucial, as is taking into account each person's unique dietary requirements and seeking the advice of medical specialists for tailored advice.

# CHAPTER NINE

# CONTRAINDICATIONS, SIDE EFFECTS, AND SAFETY

## COMPREHENDING HERBAL SAFETY

Using natural medicines and conventional medical methods requires an understanding of herbal safety. Although plant-based medicines and herbs have been used for millennia to cure a variety of illnesses and enhance well-being, it is important to recognize that they can have certain hazards. It's important to comprehend a few essential herbal safety ideas to ensure safe consumption.

The fluctuation in the strength and purity of herbal products is a major factor in herbal safety. Herbal remedies, in contrast to pharmaceutical medications, frequently have inconsistent dosages, which can affect both their safety and efficacy. The concentration of active chemicals in plants is affected by various factors, including soil quality, cultivation techniques, and climate. These factors can be responsible for this fluctuation. Because of this, people who use herbal medicines need to be cautious, start with tiny doses, and pay close attention to the results.

## INTERACTIONS BETWEEN DRUGS

The possibility of drug interactions is a crucial component of herbal safety. Similar to pharmaceutical medications, herbal therapies can have pharmacological effects on the body. This implies that they may interact with over-the-counter and prescription drugs, either increasing or decreasing their effects or resulting in negative side effects. For example, a variety of drugs, such as blood thinners, oral contraceptives, and antidepressants, can interact with herbs like St. John's wort. People who use herbal treatments must provide this information to their healthcare practitioners to prevent possibly harmful interactions.

# INTOXIOUS REACTIONS

Moreover, allergic reactions are another risk associated with herbal safety. Even though herbs are natural materials, some people may nevertheless experience allergic reactions to them. Herbal allergies can cause gastrointestinal issues, skin rashes, swelling, itching, or breathing difficulties. Thus, before beginning any new herbal remedy, people should be aware of any pre-existing allergies and, if in doubt, get tested for allergies. Furthermore, some herbs might interact adversely with allergens, making things more difficult for people who already have allergies.

## PARTICULARS TO BE AWARE OF IN HERBAL MEDICINE

The possibility of contamination and adulteration of herbal products is another special consideration in herbal treatment. Pesticides, heavy metals, or other hazardous materials could contaminate herbal supplements due to the absence of regulatory monitoring in the sector. Furthermore, some herbal products could contain illegal ingredients or synthetic medications in their adulteration. Customers must select reliable suppliers and brands that follow quality and safety guidelines because of these factors.

Anyone thinking about using herbal medicines needs to grasp the importance of herbal safety. It entails appreciating the variation in herbal goods, being mindful of possible drug interactions, protecting oneself from allergic responses, and keeping an eye out for contamination and adulteration. People should always reveal their use of herbal medications and any possible adverse effects they may encounter to healthcare experts who are informed about herbal medicine to ensure the safe and efficient use of herbal medicines.

# CHAPTER TEN

# CONTROL AND QUALITY GUARANTEED

## HERBAL PRODUCT QUALITY AND PURITY

When it comes to guaranteeing the security and effectiveness of herbal medication, the quality and purity of herbal goods are crucial. The qualities and traits of a herbal product that establish its overall medicinal potential are referred to as its herbal quality. The botanical identification of the plant, the presence of active ingredients, the lack of pollutants, and the application of sound agricultural and collection procedures are all factors that affect the quality of herbal remedies. On the other hand, purity is a quality attribute that deals with the lack of contaminants, adulterants, or other undesirable materials from herbal remedies.

Herbal product quality control encompasses a range of procedures, including chemical profiling, microbiological testing, and botanical identification, to ensure and evaluate product quality. Techniques for growing, collecting, and storing herbs correctly are essential to maintaining their quality. Furthermore, maintaining consistency in the quality of herbal products is facilitated by the use of quality assurance methods and standard operating procedures. Guidelines for determining and guaranteeing the quality of herbal products are provided by several pharmacopeias, industry standards, and regulatory bodies.

## HERBAL PRODUCT CERTIFICATION AND LABELING

To inform customers about the contents, intended usage, and safety of a product, labeling is an essential part of the process. To tell customers about the identification, contents, dosage, and usage guidelines of a product, proper labeling for herbal products is crucial. Labels should also include information about possible interactions with other drugs, contraindications, and side effects. Healthcare professionals need this knowledge to guarantee the safe and efficient administration of herbal medication, and consumers need it to make educated decisions.

One important component of quality control is the certification of herbal goods, which frequently takes the form of Good Manufacturing Practices (GMP) certification. Manufacturers of herbal products are required to adhere to GMP standards to guarantee a constant level of quality and safety. Regulatory agencies' or independent groups' certification increases customer confidence that the herbal items they buy adhere to strict quality and safety guidelines. Additionally, it gives producers that can show that they are dedicated to making premium herbal goods a competitive edge.

# LEGAL AND REGULATORY ASPECTS OF HERBAL MEDICINE

The laws governing herbal medicine are complicated and differ between nations. Herbal items are often regulated as traditional medicines or nutritional supplements in several regions. Herbal items may occasionally come under the purview of health agencies in charge of drug regulation. The purpose of these legislative and regulatory structures is to guarantee the efficacy, safety, and quality of herbal remedies.

Regulatory organizations, like the U.S. The European Medicines Agency (EMA) and the Food and Drug Administration (FDA) have set rules and regulations for the marketing and registration of herbal products. Manufacturers are required to present data on the quality of their products as well as proof of safety and efficacy from clinical trials. Strict rules also govern the labeling and advertising of herbal products to prevent deceptive or fraudulent claims.

Laws that seek to stop the exploitation of indigenous populations and guarantee just recompense for traditional healers have safeguarded traditional knowledge and cultural traditions about herbal medicine in many different countries. Herbal medicines that are based on traditional knowledge may also be protected by intellectual property rights, such as patents and trademarks.

A comprehensive system that protects the use of herbal remedies includes interrelated elements such as herbal quality and purity, herbal labeling, and certification, and the legal and regulatory aspects of herbal medicine. For consumer health and the legitimacy of herbal medicine as a treatment option, the quality and safety of herbal products must be guaranteed.